CELEBRATING THE YEAR OF ME!

TABLE OF CONTENTS

Introduction

INTRODUCTION

It's finally here! This is the year we celebrate losing weight and reaching the finish line. This is the year we shine! A long time in the making, but finally, after all the times of trying and failing, today is the day! Today we start on that journey to get to the size and weight we have always dreamed of. We WILL lose weight this time! We WILL see that bathroom scale smile at us instead of grunt and groan. The goal is within reach. Too much is at "steak" for us to quit now. We are sick and tired of being sick and tired.

We all know that being overweight is serious. Extra weight causes health problems. It contributes to heart disease, stroke, diabetes, and cancer. Losing that excess fat may be all that is needed to get off those meds and back on track. We want to look better and feel better. No matter what the reasons are, we can be confident that it can be done. Whether it's a lot of weight or not so much, we have the choice to do something about it. Today we are making that decision. Let's do it! If you've got more than 100 pounds to lose – or less, you're not alone.

So, say "Goodbye" to the big sized clothes! Say "So Long" to the huffing and puffing, trying to get up the stairs. And "Hello" to looking good and feeling great again!

This book is intended to be an encouragement to all who are trying to lose weight. I am not endorsing a diet plan. There are so many options available. It is ultimately up to you to choose which one is right for you. I have included samples to give you an idea of where to start. Whatever you decide to try, get a checkup from your doctor and take that first step. You will make it to the finish line this time. The person that succeeds is the one that keeps on trying.

STARVING IS OFF THE TABLE

We can lose weight without being hungry all the time. Some folks are reluctant to start a weight loss plan because being hungry is not fun. It's discouraging to think that to take it off and keep it off we are always going to be famished. What if we love food and hate the thoughts of having to eat carrot sticks and lettuce to make the weight come off?

Here's some good news! Starving is "off the table!"

Naturally, we have the urge to eat when we are hungry. Hunger is our signal that our fuel tank is empty, and we need to fill it up or we are not going anywhere. It can also be an indication that we need food now to avoid the danger of getting sick. So, self-preservation kicks in and we eat everything in sight to keep from starving. But you don't have to go hungry all the time to control your weight. Sticking to a healthy eating plan for regular meals will help us lose weight and feel full while we reach our goals.

Though we live in the modern world where food is plentiful, our body doesn't know that or care. It runs on instinct, going into survival mode to protect us from dying from starvation. So, for some, giving up before getting started, is better than starving. We like to eat, so being constantly hungry all the time is not an option. What fun is life if our stomach is always growling? It's not fun! It's embarrassing!

Surprise, surprise, some plans will let us eat food and still lose weight. No kidding! They are out there. We must find one that we are comfortable with and get going!

That is what we are planning to do. With enough information, we can map out a plan and set our goals. We must learn what works and what doesn't. Information is the key.

Those ugly pounds affect our self-esteem, too. We can't paint all the mirrors black, it's just not practical. Besides, we will WANT to see our new image. We may want to install more mirrors when that goal is reached. Who better deserves to look good and be healthy than we do?

We are valuable in this world. We deserve to be healthier. Excess weight that is holding us back must go. It is in our power to do something about feeling frustrated, out of control, unhappy, and miserable. This time we can win without going hungry! Gathering the tools and learning how to use them will be our first step. Our game plan starts with deciding what plan is right for us, then setting our targets within the time frame that works best for our lifestyle.

FADS? DO THEY WORK?

Weight loss and diet programs are a multi-billion-dollar business. Ads are everywhere. You are always hearing and seeing ads for weight loss products that promise miraculous results. Many are meal plans, others are pills that claim to do the impossible like burn fat and get you skinny in a week. Some others tell you that certain foods must be completely cut out of your diet to rev up your body's metabolism.

Some prepackaged programs have amazing successes, but there is a downside. They can get expensive. Some charge a membership fee, plus the cost of food. However, there are some positive things to say about the prepackaged plans. They are convenient and easy to follow. Some of them offer advice and a support line. Most will offer some encouragement when you have questions or need a positive uplift to attain your goal. It is one way to go about losing the weight that you want to lose.

 The foods are already measured for you. It is so convenient to have it delivered right to your door, instead of having to go shopping, read labels and count it all up yourself.

 You can choose to join a program if you want to. And I say, go for it! If that's what works for you, great! But if you can't afford an expensive program, you can do it all on your own. You can shop for the right foods, make your menus, and follow your plan, without spending an arm and a leg. You can learn to cook meals for yourself. We know that to lose weight we must eat fewer calories and exercise more, but we want a quick fix, so we tend to resist that idea. We want it to be fast, easy and painless.

We know what we want. To lose those extra pounds, right? Right! Of course, there are many ways to go about it. The tried and true methods will usually work better than the new miracle pill or the unbelievable skinny-in-a-bottle plan. Some of the fads are so outrageous that they are laughable. Anyone with a brain knows that it can't be done in a few days or weeks. Food choices, portion control, and an exercise routine are all things to consider when starting on this new trek.

DIET PILLS

Diet pills, to me, are a no-no. They are dangerous and most of them don't work anyway. They are made from who knows what? We know some have a lot of caffeine and other appetite suppressants. They may claim to increase your metabolism to burn fat, making you feel full. Some claim to block your body's absorption of fat. And then some are merely diuretics. You lose water instead of fat. Don't take diet pills without a doctor's approval, if you must take them at all. They can interact with other medications, too. Diet pills can be highly addictive, so know that before you start on them. Be very cautious. The right foods will give you the same effect as the fat burning pills do, and much safer. If you are determined to try them, you should be aware of symptoms that may occur.

Stop and consult your doctor if you experience anything unusual, such as symptoms like these:

High blood pressure

Heart palpitations

Fever

Anxiety or nervousness

Tightening in your chest

Irritability

Dry Mouth

Constant headache

Insomnia, restlessness, or hyperactivity

Blurred Vision

Sweating

Dizziness or any other abnormal occurrences

Diet pills are easily bought over the counter, so be careful about following the directions. Don't take more of them than is recommended thinking that it will work faster. They can be very addictive and powerful. There is a danger of overdosing if not taken correctly.

There are much safer ways to lose weight than taking pills. They did not work for me. If you choose to try them, do so cautiously and check with your doctor. Many people think they can eat whatever they want when they take these pills, but that's just not the case. If you never make any changes, you will keep seeing the same results.

Exercise, diet and lifestyle changes make all the difference. Pills are only a temporary fix and you will likely gain it all back.

I don't recommend diet pills. Pick a safe way to lose weight. It's up to you to find the one right for you. Get all the information that you need before you start. I hope this book will give you the confidence to try those other ways for yourself. I have included some ideas to help you make it a success. Let's discover what is true about losing weight and what is not.

We can examine some of the most common untruths and try some great new recipes while on this journey. Do your homework. There is a sensible plan that will work for us, one that we can be comfortable with. We can spend lots of money trying to find a quick fix. It just doesn't happen! We should know what we are doing before we start. Let's make sure our plan will balance out what our body needs to create energy and operate smoothly.

CAUSES OF OBESITY

Why are we all so fat? That's a good question. One obvious answer is fast food, but it's more than that. I'll admit that it's so convenient to stop by the restaurant and pick up a ready-made meal. It's easy to fall into that rut. Driving up to the drive-through is so much faster than shopping, cooking and counting calories and carbs. And these fast food shops are everywhere. Drive down the street and you will pass several that have been painted just the right colors to lure you in to buy the specials. The smells are not helpful, either. If we are already hungry and get whiffs of some of those delicious cooking odors, well, that battle is lost. The presence of these restaurants certainly does not help. The menus are loaded with cholesterol, fat, and calories. Check out some of the interesting documentaries about the effects of these foods and you may just decide that the convenience is just not worth the price of your health that you will eventually pay. I recommend watching some of those videos if you need further convincing. You might just have a change of heart.

There is a trend now at a lot of restaurants to offer a healthier menu. People have become more health-conscious and are demanding better choices. Some now offer salads, grilled meats instead of fried, and baked potatoes instead of French fries. At least you now have a better choice if eating out is one of your favorite things to do. Be diligent and count everything until you achieve that goal, then you can relax a little and splurge sometimes. Choices, that's what the answer is; it's all about what we choose.

It takes effort and planning to shop and prepare the best healthy menus for our families while working and doing all the everyday things that have to be done. Often, we buy the convenience of prepackaged foods that contain a lot of fat, salt, and preservatives.

All these factors add to our weight problems. Some of us are tired and just want to get home and sit down in front of the television after dinner. We have become inactive and sedentary. Few people go for long walks in the evening as folks did in the past.

Kids pick up on this same behavior. They seldom play outside the way kids used to. It used to be kickball or hopscotch; jumping rope, skating, or riding bikes. Television used to be part-time. Now kids spend more time on the computer, tv or playing video games. It's not all bad. Some programs are educational. It just seems that we are not moving enough. It would help a great deal to get up and get walking or dancing instead of sitting, eating snacks and drinking sugar-rich soda.

METABOLISM

Do you know how your weight is linked to your metabolism? I didn't. It seemed so confusing. It's not that hard to understand.

Metabolism is the biochemical process by which your body converts what you eat and drink into energy by combining calories in foods with oxygen to release the energy you need. Balance calories that you consume with those you burn, and you can lose weight. Eat more calories than you need, and you gain more weight. Eat less and you can lose it. Metabolism burns up these calories. It regulates your energy level. As we get older, it slows down because our needs change.

True, our metabolism slows down as we age, and we must adjust to it. Our exercising and eating habits must change to maintain our ideal weight, but it is something we must deal with. That's the reality of life. We must adapt to it, and we can.

Now that we know how it works, we are motivated and determined to make it this time. We have our minds made up and there is no changing it. Are you with me? Say "Yes."

ATTITUDE

We don't like to have to give up anything. We resist starting new things because of fear of failure or worrying that we can't do it. Well, fear and worrying won't help. The right attitude is important. We know that things don't happen overnight, that it takes time to develop new good practices and replace the old bad ones. We must make a conscious decision to behave differently.

I have heard that if you repeat a task for three or more days, it becomes a habit. I guess that's true. If it is, we can change our lifestyles and create new habits that will help us reach the reward that awaits us.

Let's keep our eyes on the prize. The specifics will become clearer. Focus on the big picture and don't let the fear of failure hold you back.

After all, losing weight should be easier these days with all the plans and programs in place. Getting started is hard, but it gets easier as we learn the routine.

The bad news is that it does take a lot of effort. We must pay attention to our strategy and keep track of our progress. The good news is that there are some things that we can do to put ourselves in the right mindset. It will be well worth it, I promise.

Now that we have made up our minds, let's get the tools needed to get the job done. We can learn the rules of the game and understand the basics. Let's get motivated and committed to the job at hand. We won't be distracted or tempted to turn aside. Well, if we do, we get back on track immediately. So on with the program! Let's get excited and have some fun. This new lifestyle will be ours forever. Our goal is just around the corner. We will see it through. Healthy, energetic days are ahead.

The things worth doing are never easy. It takes some willpower and grit, but we have come too far to back down now. The goal post is in sight! There is a new suit or a pair of jeans with our names on it waiting at our favorite store. No, it won't be easy, but the rewards will be worth it. Losing weight and getting our health back is a goal that we can reach. It's not rocket science!

SOME THINGS TO DO TO HELP FOCUS:

1. Grab a notebook or journal and write down what you want for yourself. It does not matter how outrageous it may be. It's your list; no one else must see it. Put on paper the goal weight that you are aiming for. Paste a picture of yourself when you looked your best on the front page of your notebook.

2. Give yourself time to accomplish your goal but set a deadline. Do it by your next birthday, or Christmas or vacation time. Mark it on the calendar. Add up how many weeks it is until the event and make it your goal to lose 2 or 3 pounds a week till that date.

3. Read over these goals every day. Make notes. Focus. Remember, these goals are important because you are important. You deserve to win!

4. Commit to keeping up the plan. Make it a priority. If you do, you are well on your way to making it to the finish line.

5. Do not get discouraged! It didn't pile on overnight and it won't come off overnight. It takes time. Cut yourself some slack.

If you take things one step at a time, there are basic strategies that can be learned. Stop telling yourself, "I just can't do it." You can coax yourself into a new habit of healthy eating. Be the Little Engine: "I think I can, I know I can!" Reach for the sky, if you miss it, you could get an eagle. Push for the prize. We have the force of power in us to achieve those dreams!

LET'S DO IT!

There are many plans available for losing weight without starving. Taking it slow and sensibly changing old habits and lifestyle is ultimately the best route to take. If we take it off slowly, we are less likely to gain it back. Most can agree on drinking a lot of water. It keeps us hydrated. Coffee, tea, and cola don't count as our water intake. Drink at least eight 8-ounce glasses of water in a day. We will learn to like it. Add a wedge of lemon or lime to make it even better.

Drinking a glass before meals will suppress our appetite some and we will not eat as much. Water does not cause weight gain. Don't skip meals. Keep it balanced. Carbs and proteins are fuel and keep us going. Always eat breakfast. Be creative and fill your plate with lots of different colors of vegetables and fruits. Remember the food pyramid of the basic food groups.

No matter which plans you choose, you will still need to increase your physical activity to lose weight. Exercise burns calories. A good workout plan is necessary if you want to succeed.

Get motivated to exercise. The key is to get moving. Find something that you can live with and get going.

So now we have a plan and an exercise routine, get out the sneakers, put on the joggers and let's get going.

EXERCISE

I don't like to exercise. It's boring and hard work. I like to do projects that keep me interested and moving. Gardening is a good example. When working with plants, time flies and it's hardly noticeable that it is a workout. Small home improvement projects are fun, too. Painting a room or adding a screened-in area will keep you busy. You will hardly notice that you are exercising.

What do you enjoying doing? How about golfing or swimming? Tennis or bike riding are great ways to exercise and have fun too.

There's no need to go overboard. Thirty minutes, three times a week will make a big difference. Do more if you like but start slow and work up to it. Be kind to yourself. Remember, it took a while to gain it, so it will take a while to lose it, too.

If you prefer to work out with a group, then go for it. Aerobic classes can be fun. Water aerobics is easy on your joints. The goal is to get your heart pumping and burn off those calories!

 There may be a benefit to early morning exercise. I'm not a morning person, but no matter what time of day you choose, be consistent. Do it every day or every other day and stay at it. It won't help to exercise once or twice a month. I tried that. It doesn't work.

It's an individual choice. Whether you want to play the old DVDs or tapes, spend a lot of money on a treadmill, or just put on some music and dance in your living room or kitchen, the important thing is that you do exercise. Walking is one of my favorites.

WALKING, MY FAVORITE!

There is something about walking out in the fresh air that is so enjoyable. If you take the time to notice the flowers, birds, and nature, it is very pleasant. Walking with a buddy makes time fly by. You hardly notice that you are getting a workout when you are talking to a friend. Walk with your dog.

Walking is aerobic, so you will be burning calories while enjoying a good brisk walk. If you can increase your walking time, the weight will come off faster, but not everyone can spend an hour. Just do as much as you can and feel comfortable with it. Learn to enjoy it. Think of it as fun, not a chore.

If you like to shop, that's a great way to get in a good walk. You are not aware that you are exercising, while you browse in the store. It all counts; shopping, cooking, washing dishes, mowing the yard, and even doing the laundry! If you are moving, you are exercising.

FOODS TO EAT AND TO AVOID

So how do we choose the right foods?

Fruits and vegetables are at the top of the list. They are low in calories and high in many vitamins and minerals. The fruit is scrumptious and filling. Beans and lentils are very filling and contain a lot of fiber. Popcorn is good for snacks. Just be careful how much butter and salt are added to it. Chips are high in calories and we usually eat a lot more than we intend to. If you crave salty or sweet snacks, have a little. Don't deprive yourself or you will eat them eventually, plus a lot more. Eat five or six small meals a day, if possible. This will help you stay full and not feel like you are starving.

 Convenience food, such as pre-packaged, are filled with sodium and preservatives. It's best to stay away from them. If you don't know what an ingredient is, it's probably not good for you. Whole grain bread and brown rice are better than white bread and rice. Stick to whole grain pasta, too.

Cut back on the caffeine, sugar and sugar substitutes. Go for naturally sweet whenever possible. Honey is great in hot cocoa or tea. Chocolate has magnesium. Just be careful how you sweeten it. Wean yourself off sodas and diet sodas. Since you need to drink a lot of water to lose weight, try water with a slice of lemon or lime in it. It can be very refreshing and very satisfying!

Use alcohol in moderation. A glass of wine or a beer is okay occasionally, but it will put on the pounds very quickly. The beer diet doesn't work. (Sorry about that!)

Before you start, clean out the refrigerator and the cabinets. Give edible foods to your local food bank. Get rid of all the temptation.

SHOPPING FOR GROCERIES

Online shopping works best for me. I can compare the prices at different stores and read the labels on the computer screen. Our local stores have amazingly convenient pick-up services.

Make a list. If you use the online service, your favorites will be saved in your account. Download the app and you can shop on your phone. This way, you are not tempted by the junk foods conveniently placed near the checkout counters. You won't be tempted to buy foods because you forgot to eat before going to the store, either. Make your plan and stick to it. Read the labels and know the calorie, sodium and carb content before you buy them.

 By cooking your meals, you won't have to buy expensive pre-packaged, boxed meals that are loaded with preservatives, calories, carbs, and sodium. You can control the salt, sugar and other spices that go into your foods. They will be less expensive and taste better, too. Eating good food will give you energy, but you will have to get moving if you are serious about losing weight.

COUNT THE CALORIES

You can find a 30-page alphabetical calorie, carb, and fiber list by searching for the USDA calorie chart on the internet. Print it, or just save it as a pdf and refer to it when in doubt about the calorie count. Lots of other information can be found there, as well.

Be sure and read the labels. Measure out the portion sizes.

Consuming fewer calories than you burn is the key to losing that excess weight. Plan your meals with that in mind.

HEALTHY FOODS TO INCLUDE:

Carbohydrates:

Beans, Lentils

White and Sweet Potatoes

Vegetables (frozen or fresh)

Corn

Rice

Fruit

Quinoa

Whole Grain Bread

Oatmeal

Tortillas

Fats:

Avocado

Seeds

Oils (olive, coconut, walnut, flaxseed or sesame)

Nuts

Nut Butters

Dairy (milk, cheese, etc.)

Protein:

Turkey, Beef, Chicken, (broiled, grilled, or baked)

Eggs

Cheese

Fish

Yogurt

SAMPLE GROCERY LIST:

Fruits: Grapes, bananas, apples, oranges, peaches, pears

Vegetables: Fresh or frozen: kale, spinach, cabbage, carrots, olives, onions and celery, garlic, radishes and broccoli, white and sweet potatoes

Berries: blueberries, strawberries, blackberries, raspberries

Grains: Choose whole-grain loaves of bread and pasta, oatmeal

Nuts: walnuts, pecans, cashews, almonds, Brazil nuts

Legumes: beans, lentils, peas

Seeds: pumpkin, sunflower, seeds

Meats: chicken, ground turkey, beef

Fish: tuna, salmon, sardines, trout mackerel, shrimp

Diary: eggs, cheese, Greek yogurt,

Oils: olive, walnut or coconut

Seasonings: sea salt, pepper, cinnamon, turmeric, oregano, basil, red wine vinegar, etc.

SAMPLE MENU FOR DASH DIET

Breakfast
1 Whole-wheat bagel
1Tblsp. unsalted peanut butter
1 Cup orange juice or 1 orange
1 Cup fat-free milk
Coffee decaf

Lunch
4 Cups kale and spinach salad/vinaigrette dressing
1 Apple (sliced)
½ Cup carrots (sliced or shredded)
Almonds & 10 wheat crackers (no salt)

Dinner
Beef and vegetable soup (Homemade)
1/2 cup brown rice
1/2 cup fresh green beans, steamed
1 medium cornbread muffin
1 cup berries
Iced tea (decaf)

Snack
1 cup fat-free, low-calorie yogurt
Trail mix with raisins & sunflower seeds
1 Cup milk (fat-free)

Breakfast
1 Bran muffin
1 Tsp. unsalted butter
1 Cup light Greek yogurt
1 Cup chopped berries, fruits, apple, avocado, and banana. 1/3
Top with nuts and seeds (walnuts, pumpkin, sunflower)
1 cup low-fat milk
Green tea

Lunch
Chopped cooked chicken burrito
1 Cup salad with green onions, celery, kale and spinach
Vinaigrette dressing / 1 Cup low-fat milk

Dinner
1 Cup cooked whole-wheat spaghetti
Garden marinara sauce
Salad with greens, orange, berries, and onion
Your favorite low-calorie dressing
Whole wheat bread, dipped in olive oil (optional)
Water with lemon or lime wedge
Snack
Granola trail mix
1/4 cup raisins
Nut pieces
Sunflower seeds

SAMPLE MENU FOR MEDITERRANEAN DIET

Breakfast
1Cup Greek yogurt
½ Cup blueberries
1 Cup oatmeal
Decaf coffee
Snack
Olives & nuts
Lunch Whole-grain sandwich with vegetables (lean protein such as egg salad or turkey)
Dinner
4oz Chicken breast (baked or roasted)
1 Cup zucchini
Salad
Breakfast
Omelet with veggies, tomatoes and onions. A piece of fruit.
Lunch Tuna salad
2 Cups green salad
Vinaigrette dressing

Dinner
Broiled salmon or grilled chicken served with brown rice and
vegetables.
Tea with lemon

DO IN ADVANCE

Planning will make it easier to stay on track. Here are a few
things you can do ahead of time to make it more convenient:

Cook beans, lentils, rice, quinoa, or pearl barley according to
directions, drain and flatten out on a cookie sheet and freeze.
Break up in pieces and store in a freezer bag in the freezer for
up to three months. Take out as much as you need for soups,
stir fry, or other recipes. Toss it into the pot or just thaw in a
microwave when ready to use. Store bean soup in a separate
container or discard. This will eliminate the need for canned
beans full of sodium.

Make a pot of soup or stew once a week and freeze in portion
size containers to save time when in a hurry or to take for lunch.
Use a microwave-safe cup.

Wash and cut up fresh vegetables for salads and store in airtight
bowls until ready to eat.

Make muffins, biscuits, frittatas or burritos ahead of time and
freeze individual servings.

Boil eggs or use egg-lets and store in the refrigerator for up to
one week.

Cook chicken, ground turkey or beef. Cool and cut up. Freeze for
up to three months. Take out portions as needed for recipes.

Buy frozen vegetables for soups and stews. They last longer than fresh, and you can take out as needed.

RECIPES YOU MIGHT LIKE

Try something new occasionally. You can succeed in your journey without starving. The variety will keep it interesting.

Eat lots of fresh fruit and vegetables.

Air Fryer Brussel Sprouts

1 bag chopped stemmed Brussels sprouts

Oil (coconut or avocado for best results)

1 Tbsps. of salt

1 Tbsps. of pepper

1 Tsp garlic powder

Preheat the air fryer to 360 degrees

Toss the Brussels sprouts in oil. Sprinkle with salt, garlic powder, and pepper.

Cook for 10 to 15 minutes or until desired crispness.

Toss after 5 minutes to cook more evenly.

Breakfast Burritos

12 large eggs

Cooking Spray

1 Cup chopped onion

1 Cup chopped celery

1 can diced tomatoes

12 Tortillas (8-10 inch)

Parchment paper cut to size for each burrito

Shredded cheese, chopped avocado, and salsa (for topping)

Beat eggs and pour into sprayed, heated skillet. Mix in other ingredients and stir. Cook until fluffy. Place tortillas on parchment paper and top with 1/12 of the mixture. Add toppings.

Fold tortilla and tuck in sides, forming a burrito. Wrap with parchment paper. Makes approximately 12 Burritos.

Freeze in a freezer bag for up to one month Heat individual burritos in the microwave until thoroughly heated.

Cauliflower Pizza Crust

4 cups cauliflower rice (buy riced or rice your own in a blender)

2 eggs

Garlic salt

1 Teaspoon dried oregano

1/2 cup grated mozzarella cheese

Preheat oven to 400.

Line a baking sheet with parchment paper and spray with cooking spray. Boil or microwave cauliflower until tender and cool slightly. Squeeze out excess water by placing in a cloth and pressing, rolling into a ball. Add all ingredients to a bowl and mix. The cheese will melt and form the crust. Press onto pizza pan and shape round or square. Bake until crispy about 15 minutes.

Cook on both sides if desired. Top with your favorite toppings. Bake another 15 minutes to cook toppings. Makes 6-8 slices.

Spicy Quinoa Soup

1 Pound lean ground beef or turkey (90% lean)

1 Cup cooked quinoa

1 Cup chopped carrots

1 Cup chopped onion

2 Tbsp. minced garlic

3 Cups chopped cabbage

1 Cup chopped fresh spinach or kale

1 Cup chopped celery

1 Cup fresh Brussels sprouts, quartered

Salt and pepper

1 Tsp. dried basil

1 Cup water

1 15 oz. can dice tomatoes

Brown the beef or turkey. Drain off excess fat. Add all ingredients and cook on medium heat for approximately 10 minutes or until vegetables are tender. Top with sour cream or shredded Italian cheese.

Cheese Omelet

3 Large eggs

Salt and pepper

½ Cup chopped onions

½ Chopped red, green or yellow peppers (I like all three)

1 Teaspoon water

1 Cup chopped kale or spinach

1 Chopped tomato

2 Tablespoons shredded cheddar cheese

Cooking spray

Beat eggs, water, salt, and pepper together. Toss kale or spinach, tomato, and cheddar in a separate bowl. Spray skillet and heat peppers and onions until tender. Pour in the egg mixture and cook eggs on both sides. Spread kale, spinach, tomato, and cheese on eggs and fold in half. Slide onto a plate and serve.

Asparagus Casserole

1 Cup French fried onions (for topping)

1 Cup shredded cheese

1 Cup cooked hash brown potatoes

2 Cups chopped asparagus

1 Tsp. salt

2 Tsp. melted butter

1 Cup chopped onions

2 Eggs

2 Cups of milk

Beat eggs, butter, milk, salt, and pepper together in a medium bowl. Fold in asparagus, onions and hash browns. Bake for 30-40 minutes until a fork inserted comes out clean. Top with cheese and French-fried onions.

Taco Salad

1 Lb. ground beef (90%)

4 Tsp. taco seasoning mix, divided

4 Taco shells

2 Cups shredded lettuce

4 Tbsps. (fat-free) sour cream

4 Tbsps. of salsa

4 Tbsps. soft (reduced-fat) cream cheese

2 Medium diced tomatoes

1 Cup (reduced-fat) shredded cheddar cheese

Water

Brown ground beef in a skillet over medium heat. Drain excess fat. Add 2 tbsp. water and 2 tsp taco seasoning mix. Simmer for 5 minutes. Remove from heat. While the beef is cooling, mix remaining taco seasoning, sour cream, cream cheese, and salsa. Toast the shells and fill shells with beef. Add lettuce, tomato, and cheese. Top with the mixture.

Easy Chicken Salad

1 Lb. cooked chicken cubed.

1 Packet ranch dressing mix

½ Cup chopped onions

½ Cup chopped celery

½ Cup oil (walnut or sesame is good)

½ Cup red wine vinegar

1 Tsp dill mustard

¼ Cup honey

Combine cooked chicken and onions, and ranch dressing mix. Add oil, vinegar, dill mustard and honey to a mason jar and mix well. Spoon over chicken and mix well. Top with croutons or French-fried onions.

Easy Pizza

1 Whole-wheat pita

1 Cup minced cooked chicken, ham or ground turkey

1/2 cup mixed bell peppers and onions (You can buy frozen)

1/4 cup pizza sauce

1/2 Sliced zucchini

1/4 cup fat-free shredded mozzarella cheese

Preheat oven to 425 degrees

Bake pita on a baking sheet. Spread pizza sauce on top of the pita. Top with sliced chicken, ground turkey or ham, peppers, zucchini, and cheese. Bake 9-11 minutes until heated through and cheese melts. Enjoy!

Cinnamon French Toast

2 Slices bread

2 Tablespoons milk

2 Large eggs

1/2 Teaspoon cinnamon

1 Teaspoon vanilla extract

12 Tbsps. of honey

Blend or whisk all ingredients except bread. Soak bread in mixture, turning once.

Place bread in a nonstick skillet sprayed with cooking spray and pour any remaining egg mixture over bread. Brown the bottom. Flip over to brown the other side.

Ham, Turkey, or Bacon Quiche

10 Strips cooked lean ham, turkey or bacon

2 10 or 12-inch Tortillas (whole wheat is good)

4 Whole eggs

1 Cup egg substitute

3/4 cup fat-free milk

¾ Cup sour cream (light)

1 Cup shredded cheddar cheese

2 Cups broccoli florets (chopped)

Preheat oven to 350 degrees. Cook ham, turkey or bacon until desired crispness. Cool.

Spray 9-inch pie pan or skillet with cooking spray. Place both tortillas in the pan (use one for thinner crust).

Whisk egg substitute and whole eggs in a bowl until blended. Mix in sour cream and milk. Crumble cooked ham, turkey or bacon into small chunks and add to the mixture. Fold in broccoli florets. Mix well. Pour into the tortilla-lined pan. Bake for 45 minutes or until filling is set. Cool and slice

Stir Fry Vegetables with Chicken and Rice

2 Lbs. mixed vegetables (fresh or frozen)

1 Lb. cooked cubed chicken breast

3 Cups of cooked brown rice

Soy sauce

Spray a large skillet with cooking spray, add vegetables. Cook until tender, add chicken. Serve on rice. Top with soy sauce.

Meat Loaf

2 Lbs. lean ground beef or turkey

3 Eggs

1 Cup chopped onion

1 Cup chopped Green pepper

1 10 Oz. can of tomato sauce

1 Cup uncooked oats

Black pepper

Ketchup for topping

Preheat oven to 350 degrees

Mix all ingredients and press into a 9 by 5-inch loaf pan or iron skillet. Top with ketchup. Bake for 60 minutes or until the center is no longer pink. Serve with green beans, potatoes or corn for a delicious home-style meal.

Ground Turkey Meatballs and Spaghetti

2 lb. Lean ground turkey

1 Cup crushed croutons or breadcrumbs

1 Egg

1 Tbsp. minced garlic

1 Cup chopped onion

1 Tbsp. dried oregano

1 Tbsp. dried basil

1 Jar marinara pasta sauce

12 Pkg. of spaghetti

1 Cup Parmesan cheese

Mix turkey, eggs, breadcrumbs, basil, oregano, garlic and onion in a large bowl. Add water if needed to moisten. Shape into 2-inch meatballs. Cook in an electric skillet or oven on 350 for approximately 15 minutes or until meat is cooked thoroughly and desired brownness. Heat marina sauce in a large saucepan. Add cooked meatballs and simmer for 15 -20 minutes.

Cook and drain spaghetti. Add sauce and meatballs to spaghetti and serve with cheese topping and French bread. Serves 6.

Chicken Noodle Soup

2 Lb. cooked cubed chicken breasts

1 Lb. whole wheat or no yolk noodles

1 Cup chopped carrots

1 Cup chopped celery

½ Cup chopped onion

2 Tbsp. olive oil

Salt and pepper

1 16 Oz. can chicken broth

1 Cup of water

1 Tsp. garlic

Sauté chopped onion in heated olive oil.

Add celery, carrots, pepper, water, and broth. Boil over high heat

Add chicken and noodles and simmer until tender. Serve with oyster crackers and cheese if desired.

CONCLUSION

Instead of eating all the wrong stuff and hanging out on the couch in front of the television all the time, we are determined to be active and eat healthier. We can do it! We don't have to listen to the media about what looks good on us. We know what size we want to be to look and feel our best. We can see in the mirror what looks good or crappy on us.

We are all different, unique.

It's a reality that we must develop new habits and get rid of the old ones. It's not easy, but it's worth it. The idea is to eat better and get moving, to make it work for us.

There is a great variety of foods that we can try while on our plan. There's no need to starve. Just change and make better choices.

If you must eat a piece of candy, go ahead. Eat just one. Try out low calorie, low carb products to see if they are right for you. Don't let yourself start feeling deprived. If you start thinking of what you can't have, you will find that you will eventually have to have it.

We have made up our minds to get rid of all that excess baggage, so therefore our attitudes must change to be successful.

We are not going for painful or sacrificial. Instead, let's try for moderation. It's up to you and me to succeed. No one else can do it for us. We have some of the tools now. We have a plan. Let's do it!

I hope this book will encourage you on your weight loss "adventure."

I have yo-yo dieted for many years; it's not healthy or fun. But this is our year to do it this time. Let me know how you are doing. Join us for encouragement, recipes, tips, etc. on our blog: Celebrating the Year of Me!

It's free!

Pick up the companion journal "The Year of Me Journal," available soon.

WEIGHT LOG

Date__________________ Weight________________

Blood Pressure__________ BMI__________________

Target Calories__________ Carbs________________

Workout Plan__________ Mood________________

Date__________________ Weight________________

Blood Pressure__________ BMI__________________

Target Calories__________ Carbs________________

Workout Plan__________ Mood________________

Date__________________ Weight________________

Blood Pressure__________ BMI__________________

Target Calories__________ Carbs________________

Workout Plan__________ Mood________________

Date__________________ Weight________________

Blood Pressure__________ BMI__________________

Target Calories__________ Carbs________________

Workout Plan__________ Mood________________

Date___________________ Weight_________________

Blood Pressure___________ BMI___________________

Target Calories__________ Carbs__________________

Workout Plan____________ Mood__________________

Date___________________ Weight_________________

Blood Pressure___________ BMI___________________

Target Calories__________ Carbs__________________

Workout Plan____________ Mood__________________

Date___________________ Weight_________________

Blood Pressure___________ BMI___________________

Target Calories__________ Carbs__________________

Workout Plan____________ Mood__________________

Date___________________ Weight_________________

Blood Pressure___________ BMI___________________

Target Calories__________ Carbs__________________

Workout Plan____________ Mood__________________

Date_____________________ Weight___________________

Blood Pressure____________ BMI_____________________

Target Calories___________ Carbs___________________

Workout Plan_____________ Mood___________________

Date_____________________ Weight___________________

Blood Pressure____________ BMI_____________________

Target Calories___________ Carbs___________________

Workout Plan_____________ Mood___________________

Date_____________________ Weight___________________

Blood Pressure____________ BMI_____________________

Target Calories___________ Carbs___________________

Workout Plan_____________ Mood___________________

Air Fryer Brussel Sprouts
Asparagus Casserole
Breakfast Burritos
Spicy Quinoa Soup
Cauliflower Pizza Crust
Cheese Omelet

Chicken Noodle Soup
Cinnamon French Toast
Easy Chicken Salad
Easy Pizza
Ground Turkey Meatballs and Spaghetti
Ham, Turkey, or Bacon Quiche
Meat Loaf
Stir Fry Vegetables with Chicken and Rice
Taco Salad

The one that succeeds is the one that never quits!

www.ingramcontent.com/pod-product-compliance
Lightning Source LLC
Chambersburg PA
CBHW051131250726
48655CB00007B/3001